# DEMENTIA EXPRESS

### Lose Your Memory in 100 Ways

### Brain Boosters Included!

## Sandeep Grewal, MD

## DISCLAIMER

This book is not intended to be taken as medical advice. Reading this book does not create a patient–physician relationship. The advice in this book is not proven by research. Consult your doctor if you have questions related to memory loss.

ISBN-13: 978-1467904285

ISBN-10: 1467904287

# TO MY MOM AND DAD

Gurdish Grewal and Atma S. Grewal

# CONTENTS

Acknowledgments        vii

1   Why and How to Read This Book    1

2   The Memory Loss Training Course    7

3   The Main Course        13

# ACKNOWLEDGMENTS

I would like to thank my patients for inspiring me to write this book, my wife Myo Marlar Nwe, MD for supporting me through the grueling task of finishing the manuscript, and my friends for reviewing early drafts and providing valuable feedback. Special thanks to:

Aye Thinzar Myo, BBA, MS Management
Myo Sandar Nwe, BE Electronics
Amardeep Grewal, MS, MBA
Sheila Rondeau, MD
David Henderson, MD
Holly Wahab, PA-C
James Y Chin, MD
Kyalsin Lin Htet
Phyusin Lin Htet

# CHAPTER 1
# Why and How to Read This Book

Gradual memory loss is rampant in our society. It is more prevalent in developed countries than in the third world. Look around you: you'll see several of your friends and family members slowly dragged toward a life of forgetfulness and ignorance. I call this process the ultimate retirement of the living brain — the senile brain.

Let me tell you how this book was written. First of all I assume that every reader of this book yearns to lose his or her memory and brain power to become forgetful. On every page I offer tips on how to lose brain power. Under each piece of dubious advice is what I call a "brain booster." These are activities you can practice in your daily life to refresh your brain and reduce the chances of losing your memory.

Why, for heaven's sake, did I write this book in such a way? Our brains pay more attention to bad advice. Good advice usually is boring and doesn't command attention. If I tell you to attend my lecture, "How to Safeguard Your E-mail," you will yawn and blink. But if I teach a class on "How to Hack into Your Friend's E-mail," you will be all ears. So this seemingly bad advice will clarify for you how people lose brain power. It is an innovative concept I devised to get the message across the barriers of the mighty brain. You can apply these concepts to understand how *not* to lose your memory. Is that not sneaky and simple?

Again this book is full of bad advice that, if followed, will make your brain dull. If you do the exact opposite, however, that means the good advice made it across the barriers of the brain. If you get confused about the right thing to do, look at the "brain boosters" at the end of each section. Dementia, a disease to define progressive short term memory loss, affects millions of people worldwide. The earlier someone gets it, the more devastating the impact. When dementia comes later in life, there is less suffering. If you do the opposite of what this book says, you can at least delay the onset of memory loss and brain degeneration—and maybe even dementia.

Is everything in this book a proven medical fact? Not necessarily. There should be no need to prove things that are logical. For example we know there is a force called gravity. We know it pulls objects down to the earth. We don't need to jump out of a plane to find out whether we'll go up or down. Logic should be respected. Asking for proof of something so logical is illogical.

It is proven that mental exercise can prevent or defer memory loss and even dementia. So by logic any activity that reduces mental exercise will accelerate memory loss in the brain. This is the concept the book is based upon.

OK! We are about to start.

WARNING! Beyond this page the tone of the book changes as if the devil himself wrote it. But we will get the message across. And you will survive.

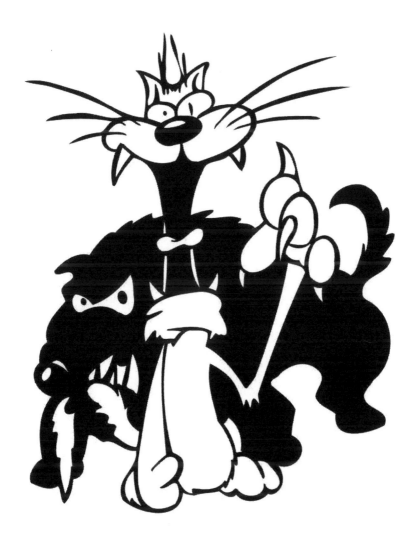

# CHAPTER 2

## Welcome to the Memory Loss Training Course

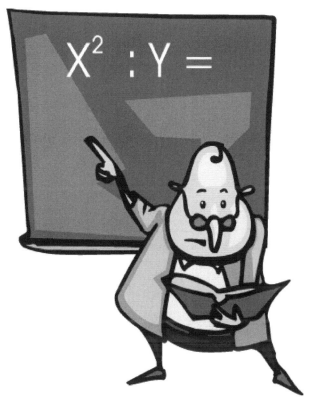

If you want to spend the latter years of your life twiddling your thumbs, with no clue where you are, this book is for you. If you'd like to achieve brain meltdown, we have several tips you can use in everyday life to meet that goal.

You might have already developed some of the habits we describe in this book. You can take it to the next level by following the rest of our advice. This way you'll develop more habits that dull your brain, especially ones you might have overlooked in the past.

There are two main concepts you need to learn before we move forward:

1. The human body is programmed to serve the mighty brain.

2. The brain is lazy and prefers to do what is easiest in the easiest way possible.

In the following sections, we will cover these two concepts in detail. Upon this solid foundation, we will add the building blocks of memory loss to turn your brain into a pudding.

## The Human Body: What Is It Programmed to Do?

Do you ever wonder what the body does all day? It makes us walk, run, see, eat, sleep, dispose, and so on. But why do our bodies have to do that? The answer is to serve the mighty brain. The sole function of the body and its various organs is to make sure the brain is alive and well. That is all a human body does—nothing more and nothing less. The human body is like a butler to the mighty brain. It caters to all its whims and fancies. The body is a hostage to the brain because it knows that if the brain does not survive, the body will not survive.

Let us go over the concept one more time. The body's sole function is to protect and nourish the brain. Everything it does is to satisfy the brain's needs, wants, and health. The body also functions to nourish and repair other parts of the body. But it does so to help these other parts provide service to the brain. For example if you get the stomach flu, your body's immune system will take care of the problem. Why? So your anorexia will go away and you can eat and digest food. Ultimately food provides nourishment to the brain. When you fall and break your arm, the fracture in the bone will heal. Why? Because with your healed arm, you can reach the food that will eventually provide nutrition to the brain. My point is that there is no other function of the human body but to serve the brain.

The body is also designed to decrease the size and function of any organ—or part of an organ—that is not needed. The body can then divert more nutrition and resources to the organs or parts that are actually working. The reverse is also true. The more you use a part of your body— the brain being no exception—the more resources are allocated to it. So if you go to the gym and start pumping iron, your muscles will get bigger. If you stop going to the gym and watch television, your biceps will shrink. Similarly if you don't use your brain - it will shrink!

# The Brain: What Is It Programmed to Do?

Unlike the body the brain is a lazy and selfish organ. It is only concerned with its survival and of course the survival of the body – otherwise it wouldn't be able to survive.

But the brain is a very clever CEO of your body. It knows how to work very little and still ensure its survival. The brain has many departments, such as: "The Talking Department," "The Listening Department," "The Socializing Department," "The Remember-the-Phone-Numbers Department," "The Remember-the-Faces Department," and so on. It continues to create more and more departments as you need them. But the brain will shut down the departments you don't use or need.

So if you don't have a phone with an address book, the brain will continue to remember the phone numbers you frequently dial. But if you decide to get that nice, fancy phone with an address book, the brain will delete the "Remember-the-Phone-Number Department" or dramatically reduce its capacity.

Why does the brain do that? It is a simple principle of management called allocation of resources. In simple terms resources are distributed to departments that actually do work and taken away from those that don't. This conserves resources and makes them last longer. This is the same way businesses work in real life.

For memory loss to come faster, we must allow the

brain to shut down as many departments as possible. We should avoid activities that stimulate the brain and keep its departments alive and functioning. With technology it's much easier now to shut down the brain. Before the advent of cell phones, we could all remember at least ten to fifteen phone numbers. But with the advent of address books, one-touch dialing, and voice-activated dialing, you might not even remember your spouse's number. We have lost the "Remember-the-Phone-Number Department."

The brain will do minimal work if you don't push it to do more. In fact every person you know will do only the minimum required work unless you push him or her to do more. That is because they all have brains! As I said the brain is the laziest of all creatures and always looks for a way out of hard work. And why did I say the brain is lazy? Every big company knows that if it makes a product that gives us an easier way to do things, it will be successful. Consider coffee shops. Is it not easier to buy a coffee than to make it? Isn't that the reason you like to go to the coffee shops?

Without further ado let us explore what we can do to make the brain dull and cloud our memories forever.

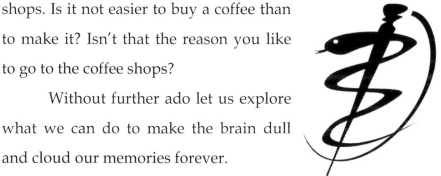

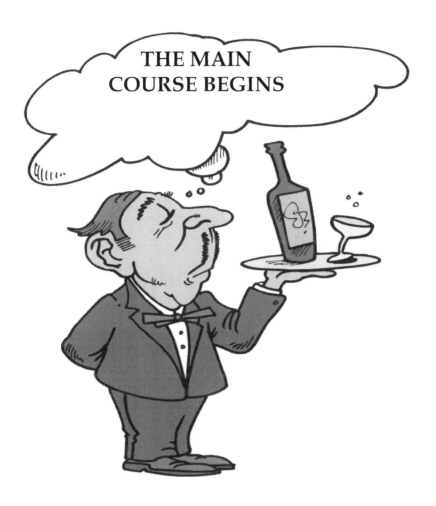

## CAUTION:

DO NOT PROCEED BEYOND THIS POINT WITHOUT

READING CHAPTER 1.

# 1. Elevator Maniac

We all love elevators, don't we? Press a button, and there you are on another floor. Most likely you start from the ground floor and go to the second floor. Life is easy with elevators. How many of us even know where the stairs are in our office building? Not many. That's why they have those big signs pointing to the stairs for us in case of an emergency. They know that we never been to the stairs.

If you haven't climbed stairs in a while, you'll notice it is not easy. You'll have to watch your step, and it will be slow at first. But if you keep climbing the stairs regularly, you might eventually skip steps and run up and down at breakneck speed without hesitation.

If you stop climbing stairs, your brain no longer has to coordinate these complex movements. When you're in the elevator, the brain just has to make you stand and stare at the wall. Anything that is easy for the brain is a formula for memory loss.

### 🕯 *Brain Booster*

*At your office, use stairs more often than elevators. Climbing up and down the stairs makes your brain practice complex coordinating and balancing movements. This is a good exercise for the lazy brain.*

## 2. Do You Hate the Riddler?

What do you do when you come across a crossword puzzle or some other puzzle in the newspaper? Listen to the inner voice saying to you, "What will I get by solving it? It looks too difficult." The tiny voice is the lazy brain we talked about earlier. It does not want to work on the puzzle because solving it will not benefit its survival. I know what you are thinking: Doesn't keeping my memory mean survival for the brain? No! For the brain, survival means living as long as possible using as little energy as possible.

The problem with doing crosswords and other mind-challenging puzzles is that it stimulates analytical thinking. And that helps the brain to grow in its capacity. So if you want to dull your brain, don't do those puzzles.

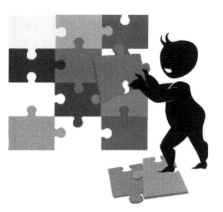

*Brain Booster*

*Doing crosswords, or any other puzzles, is a great exercise for the brain. Just like physical exercise, puzzles can be difficult at first. But the more you try, the easier it gets to solve those puzzles. Such a simple, enjoyable habit will keep your brain sharp.*

# 3. The Antisocialite

Socializing is fun, stimulating, and unpredictable. These three characteristics are enemies of memory loss. When we socialize, brain circuits whiz at lightning speed. A lot of thinking is involved in socializing. We must remember names and faces, dig up subjects for conversation, analyze other people's reactions, and so forth. The brain grows in efficiency during this activity. But that is not what you want if the goal is to lose your memory. Social isolation is an effective tool for dulling your brain. Solitary confinement has been used as a torture tool by police and military all over the world because of this effect. Many areas of the brain shut down when you avoid social interaction.

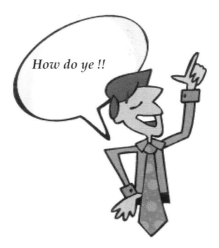

*How do ye !!*

*Brain Booster*

*Socialize with friends, family, and colleagues. It is fun and will keep your brain active and sharp. Also you won't get depressed.*

# 4. No, I Won't Do That

Always say no to anything new that is asked of you. It can be dangerously good for your memory. When we consider trying something new, we first have to decide whether it's worth the effort. We look at the options. We consider the risks and benefits. Then we have to feel the experience of trying something new. This decision-making process exercises the brain. Exercising the brain decreases memory loss. So to lose your memory, stop doing new things. Sit in the same chair, sleep at the same time, wear the same style of clothes, and eat the same foods. That should slowly dull your brain even if it does not cause memory loss.

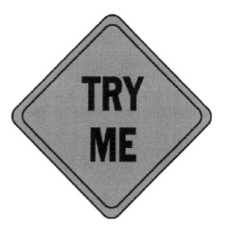

🕯 *Brain Booster*

*Always try new things. Try a new look, change the way you work, read a different kind of book, and so on. It will keep your life interesting and your brain active.*

## 5. You Can't if You Think You Can't

Run away from all challenges. Tell yourself you can't do it. When we decide to do something challenging, the brain goes into emergency alert mode. It has to reallocate resources in order to give the project a better chance of success. That's lot of work for the brain, which explains why it's so difficult to challenge ourselves. The lazy brain discourages you from accepting challenges and stepping out of your comfort zone. When we pursue a coveted job, decide to improve our golf game, or try to start a business, we challenge ourselves. That prevents us from losing our memory. So don't do it; just stay in your comfort zone. Be cozy, comfy, dull, and demented.

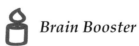 *Brain Booster*

*Challenge yourself. Always try to achieve something you believe you can't reach. On your way up, you will learn a lot of new things and become a lot smarter. You will not only avoid memory loss, but also become successful and confident.*

## 6. Think Negative

We all have goals and aspirations. Always think of something negative that will kill your motivation. This can decrease your feelings of self-worth and make you a lost soul. It is poison for the brain. You'll have no choice but to sit back and rest because all your desires are lost. When you rest, the brain rests. Too much rest and the brain will cut down its activity.

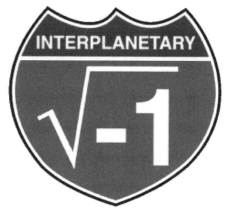

Another way to promote negativity inside you is to regularly complain about everything around you. This can be about your work, your spouse, your family, the whole world, and more. Once you become a complainer, you will not be able to do anything worthwhile, and you can be assured that your mind will rot.

### Brain Booster

*Do you have aspirations? Do you have the motivation to do something great? Then don't just sit around – do it. Get a positive attitude. Find something good in even the worst things in your life. Every cloud has a silver lining.*

# 7. TSCP — Television-Staring Couch Potato

Strive to become a dedicated television staring couch potato. Television will make it so much easier to become forgetful. Why? Television is one-way communication. All you have to do is listen. You can't argue back or have a conversation with the television. Even if you say something, 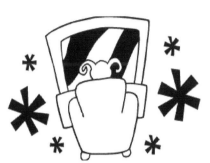 the television won't hear it — neither will people sitting with you to watch the television. Have you ever seen a middle-aged fellow sitting in front of a television, slowly wasting his life and getting older and more forgetful? I'm sure you have. Television can send people into a trance-like state. TSCPs don't even realize they're becoming demented. That's how memory loss creeps up on people who watch television for most of the day.

### Brain Booster

*Do not watch television for more than one or two hours a day. Television will put you in a hypnotic state. Never watch television in the morning; it will make you dull for the rest of the day. Treat your morning-fresh brain with something intellectual and stimulating, such as reading, exercising, or thinking.*

## 8. Burn Those Books

Don't make reading a habit. Reading a book is unlike watching television. Watching television is passive, and reading a book is active. While watching television we don't have to imagine anything at all. The sound and picture are in front of you. But when we read a book, we have to imagine the backdrop, the characters, the sounds, the mood, and so forth. Using imagination is laborious for the brain. That is one reason the brain does not like to read books.

But there is a simple, quick fix. All you have to do is stop reading books. Your imagination skills will decrease, the brain will slow down, and you will have a cool, demented brain in the vault of your skull.

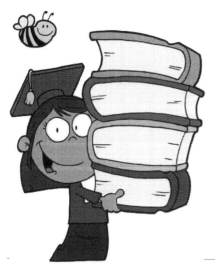

**Brain Booster**

*Read books regularly. Vividly imagine the characters, sounds, and tone. This will not only heighten the enjoyment of reading but also help prevent memory loss.*

22

## 9. One-Touch Dialing

Be friend of technology. Soon like other people you will forget they have the ability to remember phone numbers. Cell phones have made it possible to dial a number with one click. Better still, voice-activated dialing allows you to speak a name and have it automatically dialed. Who says miracles don't happen?

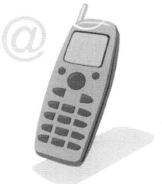

If you use this technology regularly for all your phone calls, it can effectively reduce the brain's capacity to remember phone numbers. And your dream of memory loss will be one step closer.

 *Brain Booster*

*Never use one-click dialing. Dial the whole number. Try to remember the phone numbers you dial frequently so you don't have to look them up in the address book.*

# 10. The Voice in My Car

Technology is marvelous. There was a time when we had to remember directions by heart before setting out on a trip. Or we had to navigate our way using a map. Remember when there was a Rand McNally map book in almost every car? As technology developed we began using websites such as MapQuest to find directions. With MapQuest we still had to look around to locate the streets listed in the directions. But now we have global positioning systems (GPS) mounted in our cars. Even if you don't have a GPS in your car, you most likely have it on your phone. With GPS we don't need to keep checking the names of crossroads when we drive. We don't need directions. We don't need to watch for landmarks. All we have to do is to follow the GPS voice and do whatever it tells us. Just follow commands. No need to read maps and determine north or south on our own — no thinking involved.

You don't think GPS can dull your brain? If you've been using GPS for a while, try going to a new place without it. You'll be scared to death and even doubt that you can actually do without it.

So when you go somewhere, don't try to read the map. Just switch on the GPS, and let it guide you. After all, the weary brain needs to rest in order to let memory loss flourish.

### Brain Booster

Use a GPS only if you're short on time or you're already lost. Otherwise use a map to get to your destination. Don't let reading maps become a lost art. Keep an atlas in your car.

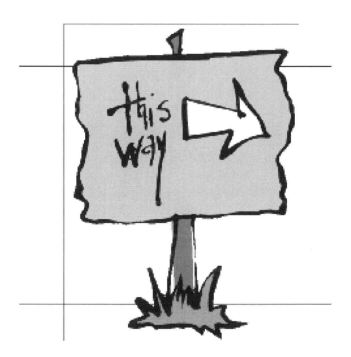

# 11. Shopping Made Simple

After checking out at the cashier I do not want you to check your receipt and add up the items. When you were on a shoestring budget in college, you might have double-checked your receipt before leaving the cashier. You didn't want to pay a dime more than needed. It was a fast check to make sure no item was charged double or more than what it was listed for. This activity can make the brain more efficient. Every time you repeat the process, it becomes faster and easier to scan the receipt. As we grow older, we do not want to put the brain through this stress.

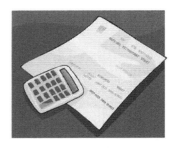

Stopping a simple activity like checking receipts can kill the circuits in the brain. Lo and behold memory loss arrives.

**🕯 *Brain Booster***

*After paying at the register, always look at your receipt. Make sure all items are charged the correct price and there are no double charges. Once you get good at it, mentally add the numbers to make sure the total is approximately correct. The habit will not only pay you back one day – it will also keep your brain active.*

## 12. The Mental Calculator

Calculations are the enemy of a brain yearning for memory loss. Nothing can save a brain from memory loss like doing calculations. Even simple everyday calculations, such as balancing the checkbook or calculating your change on a purchase, can rejuvenate the brain. So be careful not to pull

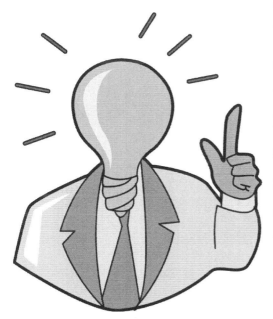

dangerous stunts like balancing your checkbook — leave it to the professionals. These little activities, which should be done regularly, must be avoided at all costs. The brain doesn't want to do the work anyway.

*Brain Booster*

*Balance your checkbooks. Calculate your change. It is all about the health of your brain, and it doesn't take much time. Don't use a calculator.*

# 13. Be a Food Junkie

Eat a lot of junk food. What is the connection between junk food and your brain? All that greasy food enters your body as fat. The fat is converted to cholesterol by the liver. The cholesterol then circulates in the blood, flowing nutrients to the body cells. Body cells are the smallest functioning blocks of the human body. Extra cholesterol starts depositing in the smaller arteries that supply these cells and blocks the flow of blood to them. Less blood flow decreases the functioning of the body cells because they cannot get enough supplies. When this kind of the blockage happens in the brain, it causes what we doctors call *vascular dementia*.

Eating junk food is key to decreasing brain functioning. It's a fun way to destroy all the powers of your brain. Sink your brain into the misery of memory loss, dullness, grease, and cholesterol—delicious!

🕯️ *Brain Booster*

*Eat fast-food no more than once a week. Try to eat healthy on the other days. Eat vegetables, low-cholesterol foods, and snacks that are less than one hundred calories.*

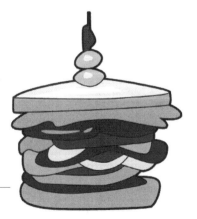

## 14. What Is Cholesterol?

Many of us do not go to our primary doctors. Many of us do not have primary doctors—and rightfully so! These doctors always try to find something wrong with us. They check our cholesterol annually and, if needed, give us medication to reduce it. If we go to the doctor for annual checkups, then 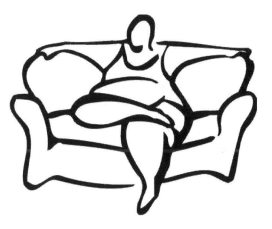 the cholesterol will not get a chance to clog the small arteries of the brain. And we will lose our chance to get vascular dementia.

Clogging the arteries in the brain can lead to strokes and cause permanent brain damage. Since brain tissue doesn't heal back, there is no treatment for this kind of memory loss.

*Brain Booster*

*Go to your doctor, and get your cholesterol checked every year. If you have high cholesterol, take your medicine and watch your diet. Keep the cholesterol levels under check so you don't clog the arteries of your brain.*

## 15. Meet Mr. Chimney

Cigarettes are friends of cholesterol. They contain agents that cause inflammation in the lining of the arteries. Inflammation helps cholesterol plug the arteries faster. That is one reason smokers tend to age faster than nonsmokers. Smoking wreaks havoc not only on our lungs but also on our heart and brain.

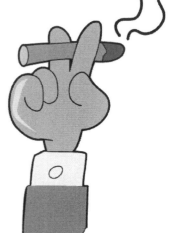

If you smoke and have high cholesterol, you have hit the jackpot for memory loss. Cholesterol will be grateful to have the support of tobacco to do what it does best: plug the arteries in the brain.

*Brain Booster*

*Don't smoke. If you already do, then stop – now! It is not worth paying money to get cancer and other horrible diseases. Did you know smokers look about ten years older than non-smokers of the same age? And it is no longer hip to smoke – it is disgusting.*

## 16. Illicit Drugs and Memory Loss

Yes, I am talking about illicit drugs. Cocaine, marijuana, heroin — you name it — are very good at destroying logical thinking. They can fry the brain like a fish in boiling oil. Illicit drugs alter the chemical transmissions between nerve endings and can affect brain functioning for a long time to come. Also drugs such as cocaine can cause a sudden spike in blood pressure, which can 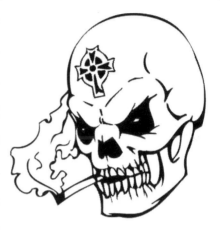 lead to strokes and heart attacks. What a way to destroy the brain!

**🕯 *Brain Booster***

*Stay away from illicit drugs. It doesn't matter how much willpower you have or how easily you can break a habit. Illicit drugs will destroy your life, relationships, and even your brain.*

## 17. I Am Heavy. Who Are You?

For your benefit scientists have proven the link between memory loss and obesity. The more you ignore the pounds, the better your chances of becoming demented. Why that happens is still a big question. Some say obesity causes inflammation all over the body, and others think it's because fat cells cause diabetes, high cholesterol, and other problems. Obesity can lead to strokes, thus damaging the brain and causing what is called *multi-infarct dementia* — memory loss due to multiple strokes. There are many different ways that fat can cause memory loss. So keep those pounds on, and do not diet or exercise if you want to get dementia.

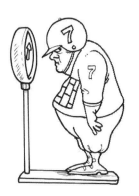

*Brain Booster*

*Diet, exercise…do whatever it takes to shed those extra pounds. Not only will you feel lighter but also smarter. It's a challenging test of willpower too.*

## 18. House Potato

There is so much to do in the house. Why should anyone leave? If you stay in the house, you can sit on the couch all day. The problem with going out is that it exposes you to new and different experiences. These new experiences

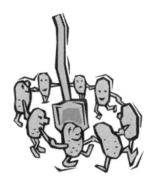

stimulate your brain much more than your mundane trips between work and home. Anything the brain does on a routine basis is not registered by the brain into new circuits; it just flows through the old circuits. So deciding to go out after work to different places can negatively affect your chances of dulling your brain. Try to avoid going to parks, museums, shopping malls, movie theaters, etc. Don't even consider going for a walk in your neighborhood.

*Brain Booster*

*Leave your house for more than just work. Go out, party, and experience life outside the walls of your house. Go to the lake, the mountains, or the golf course. Your house is nice, but the world outside is much more beautiful.*

# 19. Anti-Argumentarian

When someone talks about politics, asks your opinion, or says something you don't agree with, what do you do? Do you argue back, debate, and spark a conversation? Or do you just kill it by saying, "Uh, OK"? If you do the latter, you are doing the right thing because the memory loss will strike you faster. The lazy brain loves to just lie around and do nothing. If you have to carry on a conversation, the brain needs to work. It needs to produce verbal material and good arguments. All these activities stimulate the brain to use more neuronal circuits. Too much of this stimulation can destroy your dream—the utopia of memory loss. Next time someone asks you if Mr. President was right or wrong, just say "whatever." Don't argue.

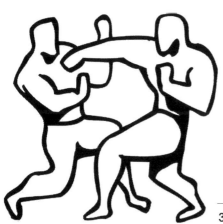

**Brain Booster**

*Argue and debate. Do not ignore conversations, but participate in them. Don't just sit in the office meeting—say something. It is good for your career and good for your brain.*

## 20. What Did You Say?

If you have trouble hearing, make sure you do not fix it. You heard it right—do not fix it. Hearing sends multiple sounds or stimuli from the environment to the brain. Some are ordinary sounds we don't even notice, but many are new and different sounds that make us go "aha." These sounds generate new circuits in the brain to register them, rejuvenating the brain in the process. If you cannot hear the sounds around you well enough, your brain will start to shut down the parts involved in hearing and sound comprehension. Losing this vital brain function will give sluggishness free reign inside your brain. Is that not what you want?

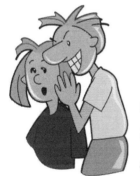

### Brain Booster

*If you have a hearing problem, go to the doctor and get it fixed. Don't just get used to it. Use hearing aids if necessary. I know they are expensive, but it's worth keeping your brain sharp and being able to hear the sounds of nature and your snoring spouse.*

# 21. Gardening Is for Gardeners

However mundane a task may seem, it can still stimulate the brain. No wonder memory loss affects people who don't do anything. Avoid gardening too. When you do yard work or gardening, your brain has to analyze the condition of the soil and plants. It then has to develop a plan to grow the plants and landscape the yard. It has to formulate the plan in steps to make sure it is efficient. This is analytical thinking. Analytical thinking is medicine for preventing memory loss and keeping your brain sharp. But that is not all. Yard work and gardening are also exercise, which is proven to reduce the chances of experiencing memory loss. So if you plan to twiddle your thumbs in your golden years with dull brain, cease all gardening and yard work now. Give up your lawn mower and hire a landscaping service. Tell them to do whatever they want with your lawn—just make it look beautiful. Maybe you will remember to notice the difference.

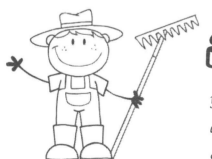

*Brain Booster*

*Do some gardening in your yard. Mow your own lawn. If you don't have a backyard, consider growing indoor plants. It is good exercise, and all that planning is good for your brain.*

## 22. You Should've Called the Handyman

Don't fall in to the trap of becoming a handyman in the house. There is always a lot of work to do at home. A light bulb needs to be changed, the garage door is not working, the bathtub needs to be caulked, etc. We have two choices — fix these things ourselves or just ignore them. Most of us don't know much about being a handyman, so we just have to figure it out. Such activities lead to learning new skills. Learning new skills is surely not the way to lose your memory. It will in fact reduce your chances of losing your memory. That is not what we want — we want memory loss!

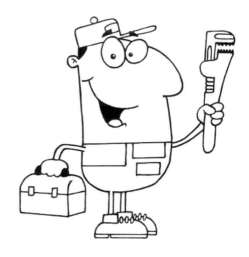

*Brain Booster*

*Fix the problems in your home. Be a handyman. Look around your house every weekend to see if there is something you can fix. Read a do-it-yourself manual or do research on the Internet. You will not only maintain your house and save money but also keep your mind sharp and your spouse happy.*

## 23. Worry, Worry, Worry

We want you to worry a lot. We want you to be stressed about everything around you. Excessive worrying increases blood pressure. High blood pressure damages the lining of the arteries in the brain. Then cholesterol will seep into the artery lining and produce blockage. Blockage will lead to strokes. So how does that help you lose your memory? If Alzheimer's is a local road to memory loss, strokes are highways to the downtown of memory loss. One big stroke or a couple of small strokes can cause sudden impairment of memory and analytical thinking. A stroke is the fastest way to dull your brain.

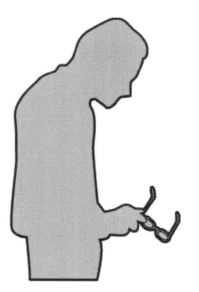

🕯 *Brain Booster*

*Don't worry excessively. Don't make it a habit. If it already is a habit, get rid of it by reminding yourself of the negative consequences whenever you catch yourself worrying.*

## 24. My Blood Pressure Is Higher Than Yours

You should not get your blood pressure checked if you want to lose your memory. Why? If you find out your blood pressure is high, you will most likely seek treatment. As I explained before, high blood pressure causes cholesterol to coat your arteries. These blockages will lead to strokes. And strokes can lead to instant memory loss. The superhighway to memory loss will be all yours.

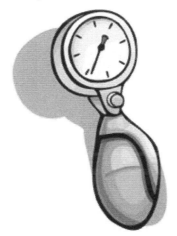

 *Brain Booster*

*Get your blood pressure checked. The top number is* systolic *blood pressure and the bottom number is* diastolic *blood pressure. Ask your doctor what the target numbers are for you.*

# 25. Keep the Doctor Away

Primary care doctors have long been focused on preventive medicine. Doctors check blood pressure and cholesterol. They put people on aspirin. Such innocent-looking medical interventions can keep you healthy. Healthy people usually do not lose their memory because their eyes, ears, lungs, heart, kidneys, etc., are taken care of. Get rid of your primary care doctor, and soon you will accumulate the kinds of medical problems that will eventually turn your brain to mush.

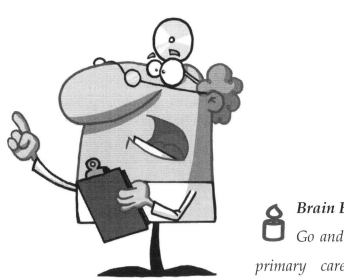

*Brain Booster*

*Go and get yourself a primary care doctor. Let them screen you for preventable diseases. Let them counsel you about your vices. Even in those short rushed visits there is a lot to learn and improve your lifestyle*

## 26. Every Day Is a Sunday

Whether it's Easter or Cinco de Mayo, aren't you bored with doing the same things over and over every single year? Why not just forget about it and sit at home bored. So what if there is a Fourth of July parade or fireworks? You don't have to be there to watch it. You don't have to acknowledge the parade on the television. Pretend it's just another day. Let there be no difference between Christmas and the day before or after. Not only will the little joys of holidays seep away from your life, but you will also become depressed and forgetful.

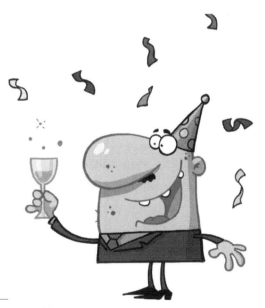

*Brain Booster*

*Keep your family traditions alive. Celebrate them with your family and pass them on to the next generations to come. Traditions give you life.*

# 27. The Writing Illiterate

Not writing everyday is a good thing for you. Why should we write? Why make the hand tired. We can always type. Many of us have not written a thing on paper since school. It gets even better after retirement. Most people stop writing after they retire except for the occasional to-do list. Nowadays we either type or don't write at all. The complex movements required for writing involve a lot of electrical impulses from the brain to control the many small muscles of the hand. This extremely delicate and precise control leads to smooth handwriting. If you think writing is easy, ask someone who has tremors.

You might ask: Isn't typing a form of writing? No! Tap-tap-tap typing is a much simpler than writing. The brain does not have send as many fine instructions to your hand as when writing by hand. Coarse movements of the hand are good enough for typing. So if you don't write, the brain responds by archiving some of the circuits needed for handwriting. As you slowly lose handwriting skills, another feather of memory loss is added to your hat.

Another issue with writing, including typing, is that the brain is forced to remember spelling—something we don't have to do while speaking. This also helps prevent the blissful effects of memory loss. If you stop writing, or even typing, the brain is happy because it doesn't have to remember how to spell, and it doesn't have to perform complex motor movements. The brain will then shrink its spelling and hand-control departments.

**Brain Booster**

*Write a page every day. Try keeping a diary or journal. The day when humans forget how to write by hand is not far away. They will only type. Don't be a part of it.*

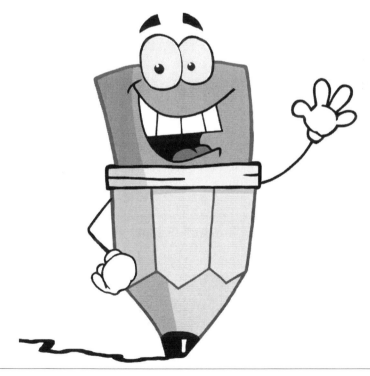

## 28. Avoid Relatives and Superlatives

Relatives have always been a problem for many of us. You can't live with them, but you can't live without them. They fight, they argue, they help, and they support. We have to remember their birthdays, keep track of their lives, help them out, and so on. Relatives keep the brain on its toes for sure. Also the feeling of being loved by relatives tends to keep the brain healthy. If you avoid your relatives and try to forget them, your brain won't have to use those circuits to keep track of them. Even the distant memories of them will slowly fade into oblivion. And don't worry — once memory loss sets in, even if they come back into your life it won't really matter.

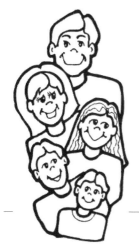

*Brain Booster*

*Check on your relatives. Make the effort to visit them across state lines. Stay in touch. If you have not seen your brother or sister in a year, there is a problem.*

## 29. Once upon a Time

We love life after retirement, don't we? When we are part of the workforce, remembering the day and date is part of the job. After all you don't want to appear dumb at work. But after retirement who cares about the date? The less you try to remember the day and date, the more the brain will rest. The more restful the brain becomes, the more rusty it will get. Soon you will only remember the month and the year. As you get better at forgetting the date, you'll probably remember the year only. Sweet memory loss is already here.

***Brain Booster***

*Always remember the day and date every single day, especially if you are already retired. Look at the calendar. Be aware of the time.*

## 30. BBCG — Belated Birthday Card Giver

Become a BBCG consistently. Why? When we were kids and teenagers, we loved to remember birthdays. We loved to surprise and impress our friends and families. We got their approval and showed our love by remembering these socially important dates.

As we get older, we no longer care about approval. We

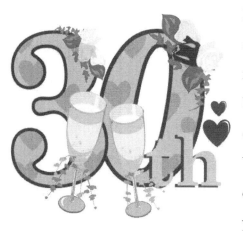

have already approved ourselves. So there is really no need to remember the birthdays and anniversaries of our parents and friends. Your spouse's birthday is a different issue. Not only can you lose your memory but also your home. I'm sure you're smart enough not to mess that up. Make it a policy that you will not remember anyone's birthday. At this point your brain will shut down the birthday recall center, and another ability of the brain goes down the drain. Hurray! One more point in favor of memory loss.

🕯 *Brain Booster*

*Remember to call and wish a happy birthday to your close friends and family. They will love you and you will stay sharp.*

# 31. Restaurant Déjà Vu

When we're in our twenties, we love to try new foods. We try Chinese, Japanese, Italian, Mongolian—you name it. We see the menu and say, "Well, that one I already had. Let me try this one." As we get older, we don't like to take chances. We go to the same restaurants that we think are good and eat the same foods. It's a great way to get rid of brain cells. You don't have to think of new restaurants to choose. You don't have to ponder the menu, read the ingredients, imagine what it tastes like, and then make a decision. That is so much work. And since you are avoiding all this intellectual work, you will be rewarded with a dull brain and the same old stinking food.

*Brain Booster*

*Go to new restaurants. Even if you are going to the same restaurant, try something new from the menu. You will be surprised and may be have a new favorite.*

# 32. Making Decisions Is Not My Forte

You don't have to make decisions. When we're kids our parents make decisions for us. As we grow up, they let us make more decisions for ourselves. The brain gets brighter and more confident when we make decisions. Move forward to adulthood, and now we make all decisions on our own. We take life in our own hands. Eventually we get married. Now we have a buddy. Why don't we just let that buddy make all the decisions? Then your better half has to do all the thinking, consider the pros and cons, and imagine the consequences before making a final decision. Making decisions for ourselves is so complicated. But your brain has to do nothing now since you've put the decision making on someone else's shoulders. As the years pass, the light in your brain will get dimmer and dimmer.

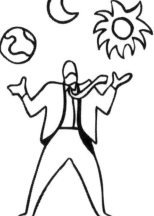

🕯 *Brain Booster*

*Make decisions for yourself, and run your own life. Don't let anyone else run it for you. If you do make a wrong decision, you can always make it right.*

## 33. The Best Retirement Is Early Retirement

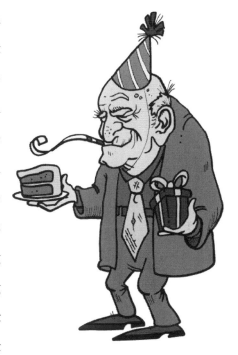

Always dream of an early retirement. Retirement is a very good way to accelerate memory loss. When you are employed, you have to be expert in whatever you do—otherwise you could lose your job. Working means remembering details, getting ready every day, deciding who to meet, deciding what to talk about, and so on. But once you retire, all that goes away. You become your own boss, and you have to answer to no one. If you forget some detail, no one will know. Gradually your brain will forget all those great abilities you acquired during your working life. That's why all those retirees around you suddenly start falling apart.

 *Brain Booster*

*Do not retire early. If anything try to retire as late as possible. Retirement is overrated.*

## 34. The Adviser Has Left the Building

If anyone asks you for an advice, give them a cold shoulder. People always ask for advice from each other, especially friends. But when you give advice to people, there is lot of brain work involved. You have to consider the circumstances, put yourself in their shoes, study the consequences, and recall your own experiences to assess the situation. It involves socializing and making friends, which electrifies the brain. But if you ignore the requests from your friends and resist the temptation to give advice, soon you won't be able to give advice at all—just like those people with dull, forgetful brains.

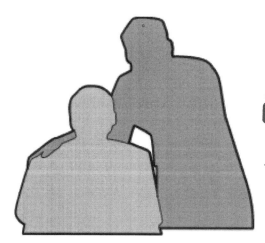

**Brain Booster**

*Listen to the woes of your friends, and advise them accordingly. They will appreciate it, and you'll never be lonely.*

## 35. The Antifriendship Band

Friends are such a hassle. Why should anyone have friends? It takes so much effort to make friends. You have to devote time to them, socialize with them, remember their birthdays, celebrate holidays with them, go to new places with them, and help them when they are sick. Just having friends can prevent depression and keep your brain active and engaged. But that is not the idea here. The idea is to keep the brain dull and depressed. So don't even try to make friends lest you end up being happy and sharp. In fact try to lose all your friends so you are confined to your house with nowhere to go. And slowly but surely your brain will lose its shine.

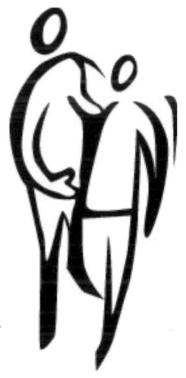

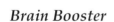 **Brain Booster**

*In life make friends — not just acquaintances. People lose the art of making and being friends as they get older. Don't let that happen to you.*

## 36. Where Is My Hobby?

Aren't you glad you don't have hobbies? We all had hobbies when we were young and single. Then along came work, family and never ending responsibilities. We got so busy that we lost our hobbies. Good riddance. Hobbies keep us hooked on a subject as we try to gather more information about it. The rocket hobbyist wants to fly the rockets higher and higher, and the photographer wants to improve his or her pictures. The only way to sustain a hobby is to read, experiment, and use your brain. That is not going to make your brain slow. A dull brain comes when you give up all your hobbies and stop learning about them.

*Brain Booster*

*Have some hobbies. Don't just do stuff for money – do things for fun as well.*

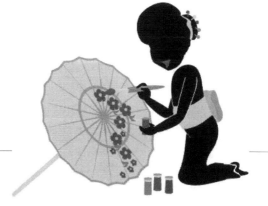

## 37. Loud Is Music

The brain is an organ that takes in information in the form of sensory signals such as vision, sound, touch, taste, and smell. Then it analyzes the information and spits

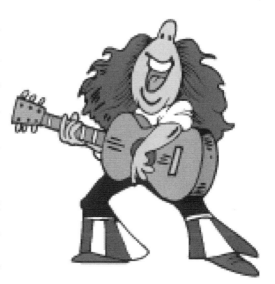

out a response. It happens fast, but it is a lot of work for the brain. If one of these incoming signals is stopped or reduced, the brain has to do less analysis. The easiest sensation to dampen is sound. All you have to do is find a way to damage your ears so you won't hear as well. The best and most fun way to damage the ears is to listen to loud music. Loud sound is a great force and can damage those sensitive and delicate filaments in your ear. Soon your hearing will decrease and your brain will work less on hearing analysis. Voila—a dull brain!

*Brain Booster*

*Protect your ears. Avoid loud sounds and music. If your work environment is loud then use ear plugs.*

# 38. Television Games: All Are Not the Same

You need to watch *Deal or No Deal, America's Funniest Home Videos,* and the like. These are good shows to watch if you do not want to use your brain. Never watch intellectual shows, such as *Spelling Bee* and *Wheel of Fortune,* which stimulate the analytical centers of your brain as you try to answer the questions before the participants do. These shows surreptitiously entice us to participate by guessing the answer before the participants do. Shows like these can actually make you smarter; they can keep your brain sharp. But wait—we don't want to be smarter, remember? So choose TV shows that do not involve mental stimulation—the kinds of shows you can watch with your mouth open and eyes glazed.

*Brain Booster*

*Choose TV shows wisely. Watch quiz shows that give you an opportunity to participate from your own living room. Avoid one-way communication shows that do not encourage viewer participation.*

## 39. Be a Staycationer

The only place you need to go every single day is your workplace. You need to stop noticing the environment around you as you drive. Now you don't have to think about how to get there. You don't notice the landmarks on the way to your work either. At work you don't

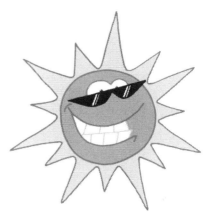

even notice what's on the shelves at work unless it has changed.

But everything changes when you go to a new city to visit. When you travel to a new place, the brain gets all kinds of new signals to analyze. The activity is no longer monotonous; the brain has to be more involved. It needs to find new roads, sources of food, entertainment, and shelter. The brain now works to assimilate all this new information so it can feel comfortable in the new place. That's why new places are not good for promoting brain dullness. Just go to work and back and you'll be on a faster track to obtaining the reward of a slower brain.

*Brain Booster*

*Travel to a new place, whether it's a new museum in your town, a nearby city, or a far-off country.*

# 40. Willpowerless

Willpower is no good for those trying to weaken their brains. Just do whatever you impulsively feel like doing. Self-control actively engages the brain because it fights against impulsiveness. Willpower is the brain's mechanism for inhibiting desires. If you drop your willpower and act impulsively, your brain does not have to gather information about your desire, analyze the consequences, and tell you whether or not to do it. It saves the brain a lot of work and makes it very lazy. Impulsiveness also decreases your self-esteem and lends itself to social isolation, which will eventually slow down your memory and your brain.

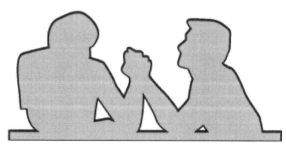

*Brain Booster*
*Have willpower and test it often. Regularly testing your willpower tells your brain who is the master — and that's you.*

## 41. Worm in a Bookstore

Let's not dare step into a bookstore or a library. What do people do in bookstores? They read. What does reading do? It prevents memory loss. There is no way we are going to enter those bookstores. Otherwise we will read and gather more information for the brain to feast on. Then the brain will use that information to develop ideas. The brain will stay active and bustling. Then we will never achieve memory loss. Avoid bookstores and libraries! Yearn for memory loss! I don't understand why are you even reading this book.

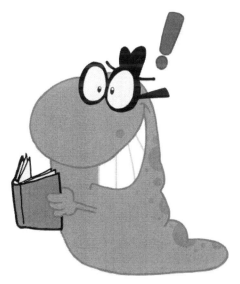

🕯️ *Brain Booster*

*Go to a bookstore at least two or three times a month. Browse books and read. Try reading something not related to your field of work.*

## 42. Be a Spectator, Not a Gladiator

Playing sports is for kids. Adults should just watch games on television. Sports are a form of exercise. It is well-known that exercise can prevent memory loss. While playing a sport, the brain has to execute strategies at a very fast pace. A sport such as racquetball makes the brain think many times faster than its usual speed. No wonder slower games such as golf are popular among adults. Don't get me wrong, even golf can dangerously improve your brain power.

Stay away from playing sports! Just watch them on television. Watching sports is one-way communication, and the brain doesn't have to think much except to remember a score here and there.

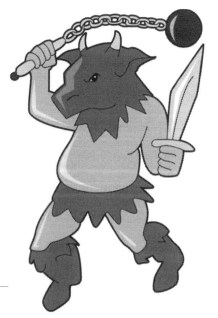

*Brain Booster*
*Play a sport and try to excel at it. Try to learn a new sport every year or two. Be a gladiator and not a spectator.*

## 43. Politics and Fashion

Shun politics and fashion, the most talked about topics in the world. Talking about such things requires the brain to do research, 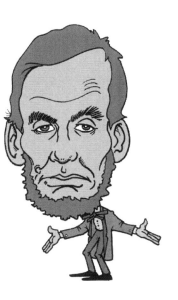 analyze information, and make observations.

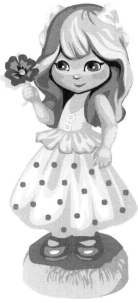

Without doing the above, it would be hard for you to hold your ground during such conversations. Ignoring politics and fashion will certainly decrease the amount of work your brain has to perform, and memory loss will creep up slowly without much notice. Simply reduce your interest in these two universal topics.

 *Brain Booster*

*Women and men of flesh and blood: read and talk politics and fashion.*

# 44. Don't Call Them — They Will Call You

Avoid calling on your friends. It is not in our best interest.

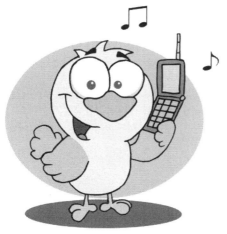

One of my friends is great at networking. He has a contact diary that he cannot live without. The diary has phone numbers for almost all the people he has met since he came to his senses. Every year the diary grows by leaps and bounds. Surprisingly he calls almost all of them at least once a year. With this determined approach, he can get almost anything done, anywhere in the world, with just a few phone calls. But this poor soul is not going to lose his memory. Networking with so many people keeps his brain sharp. Another side effect is that he is extremely successful. It is harder for successful people to lose their minds since they have so much going for them.

### Brain Booster

*You got it. Call and stay in touch with people you know. Networking is great for your career, social life and the brain.*

## 45. Develop Phone Phobia

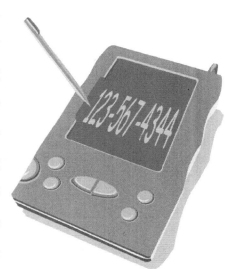

When I was growing up, the only way to find out who was calling was to pick up the phone and answer it. The pickup rate for any call coming into our home was 100 percent. Some calls were welcome and others were not, but we answered them all. That's a lot of exercise for the brain. Immediately after picking up the phone, the brain is put on the spot. It has to answer questions with little time to think.

We don't have to do that anymore. We have caller ID. We can see who is calling and easily avoid unpleasant calls. So the brain never gets stressed out and never gets exercise. If you want your brain to melt down, always look at the caller ID before picking up the phone.

🕯 *Brain Booster*

*Uncertainty of who is on the line should not scare you from picking up the phone. Don't look at the caller ID. Just pick up the phone!*

# 46. Walk the Dog, Not Your Family

We are fortunate that family walks are becoming history. Family walks were very popular back in the days when television was less pervasive. Families and their friends would go out at least once or twice a week. It was terribly good exercise and a occasion for reflection. During these walks the brain would analyze things happening in the family and then engage in discussion to find solutions to problems and plan for the future. In addition walking is an exercise known to decrease chances of memory loss.

But you do not want to prevent memory loss. You *want* memory loss. Isn't that why you're reading this book? Don't go on these walks that will make your brain sharper. Do nothing instead, and your brain will waste away. It is easy, and it is as relaxing as the walks.

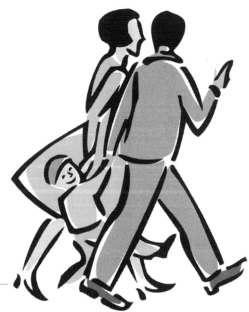

**Brain Booster**

*Go out for walks with family and friends. It will nourish your brain and also foster great relationships.*

## 47. Cold Emotions

Suppress your emotions. Don't be cool. Be cold as ice. We all experience anger, sadness, frustration, happiness, love, and so forth. But we should not express all emotions equally. Find your suppressing ability. Some people cannot express anger, while others cannot express love. Some cannot be happy; others ignore sadness and bury it in the subconscious. Expressing emotions makes the brain work harder. The brain has to decide how to express the emotion and figure out a solution for it.

If you keep your emotions suppressed, you'll get a suffocating feeling that will make you reclusive and depressed. Expressive people are usually sharp in old age. We certainly don't want that!

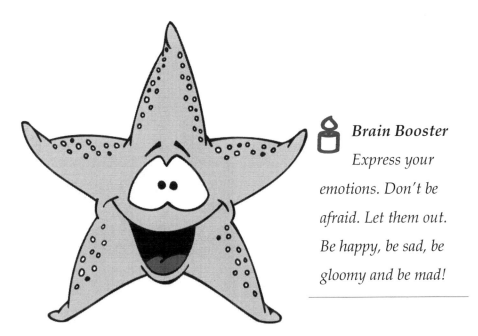

*Brain Booster*
*Express your emotions. Don't be afraid. Let them out. Be happy, be sad, be gloomy and be mad!*

## 48. Exercise Caution

Avoid exercise at all cost. Exercise has been scientifically linked to delaying memory loss. Exercise

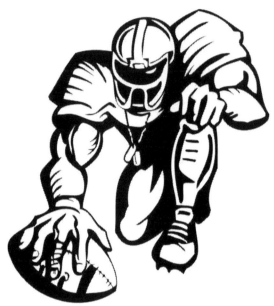

generates chemicals in the brain to improve its health. If you do not exercise at all, then your memory is probably fading the way you want it to. If you do exercise, you need to stop — otherwise your brain might stay healthy for a long time, and you will remember more than your friends and colleagues. The only exercise you should perform is exercising caution.

 *Brain Booster*

*Exercise releases endorphins in the brain which make you happy. If you exercise regularly for few months you will get addicted to it. And it is a good thing.*

## 49. Responsibility to Drink

Alcohol in large amounts can help you lose your memory faster. Alcohol depletes two vitamins in the body: thiamine and folic acid. Vitamins are necessary for normal brain functioning. Once you get rid of these vitamins, you will start forgetting things very easily. It's called Korsakoff's psychosis. In this condition alcoholics make up facts to cover their memory lapses. Alcohol can also cause seizures, which can further damage the brain. It also affects the gait 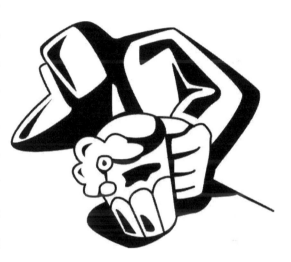 and can make you walk funny — so many bonuses just for drinking alcohol!

## 🕯 Brain Booster

*Drink responsibly. Abstaining altogether is even better if you have an addictive predisposition. For those who drink in moderation, keep it limited to red wine, not more than a glass three times a week.*

# 50. An Engine Called the Thyroid

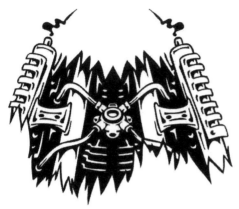

Pray to get a medical condition commonly called hypothyroidism. In this condition the thyroid gland stops producing enough thyroid hormone. Thyroid hormone is needed for metabolism—that is, the engine that runs the body. Low thyroid hormone leads to decreased functioning of the brain and other organs. It can cause a reversible form of memory loss or dementia. So make sure your doctor does not check your thyroid levels. If you do have low thyroid levels, he or she will correct it by giving you medicine, and you will lower your chances of losing your memory.

Perhaps you already have hypothyroidism and take medication for it. Rest assured that if you stop taking your thyroid pills memory loss and other problems will cloud your life.

*Brain Booster*

*Get your thyroid level checked at least once after age fifty. If you feel cold or tired all the time, then get it checked no matter what age you are. If you're already on thyroid pills, take them regularly.*

# 51. Aspirin Is a Religion

As we get older, arteries in the brain gradually narrow due to cholesterol plaques. Arteries are the pipelines of the brain that supply blood to brain cells. These cholesterol plaques can jam the whole artery and cause a stroke by stopping the blood supply to the brain. But we've already covered that. Every time someone has a stroke, a part of the brain goes dead. If someone has a big stroke or multiple small strokes, it can cause stroke-related memory loss.

One aspirin a day can prevent certain kinds of strokes. So be careful not to take aspirin if you want some good heavy-duty memory loss and strokes.

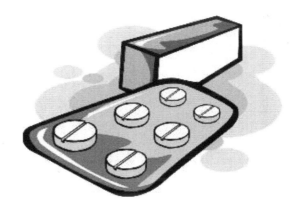

 ***Brain Booster***
*Check with your doctor to see if you should take a baby aspirin once a day.*

## 52. Being Antisocial

Don't smile at people. Don't talk to people. Never invite them to your house. Use the excuse that you're guarding your privacy. If you do invite people into your house, they will come. Why is that a problem? All these visitors will make the brain electrified and happy. There is talking, laughing, analysis of comments and gestures, and so forth. We don't want the brain to be so active — what if it gets smarter? So be aloof and uninviting. If your family entertains guests in the house, go hide in a room and do not come out until they are gone.

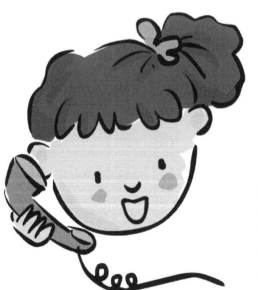

🕯 *Brain Booster*

*Get over the need for privacy. Invite people to your house. Mingle and have fun, and you'll get a razor-sharp brain in return.*

## 53. Intelligently Absentminded

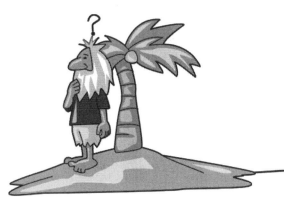

It is good to be absentminded. We can all get distracted at times. But some of us are simply absentminded. We lose our keys, forget where the car is parked, and miss important meetings. Do not correct this problem by being more observant. The less you worry about absentmindedness, the less your brain has to work. A nonworking brain will surely be a duller brain. Nothing is better than a dull, absentminded brain.

🕯 *Brain Booster*

*Don't be forgetful. Be alert about where you leave things. Consciously remind your brain what you are doing and where are you keeping things. Use associations for reminders. Shun absentmindedness.*

## 54. Down With Newspapers!

Burn all newspapers. Reading a newspaper is different from reading a book. It does several things that happen almost subconsciously. A newspaper makes you aware of the world around you. It makes you aware of the calendar date. It takes you places you have never been and helps you imagine how an event might have occurred. News stimulates debates, arguments, and critical thinking. It exposes you to new things and widens your perspective. News is food for your brain, and it enhances your opinions, creativity, thoughts, and conversational skills. All this is too much for the brain. It would rather sit idle and do nothing. For the brain being inactive is the ideal state, and one way to accomplish this is to be ignorant about the world around you.

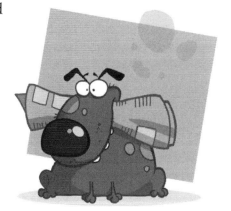

*Brain Booster*

*Subscribe to a newspaper. If you want to make your news reading productive, consider reading financial news.*

## 55. The Real Retirement

Your daily schedule is so stressful. You have to wake up early in the morning, decide what to wear, and find the fastest way to get to work on time. While coming back from work, you have to think about how to get chores done when you get home. But after retirement there is plenty of time. Why ruin it by volunteering or doing post-retirement work? Work and volunteering will put your life back on a schedule. Then you will have to do more thinking. Thinking only makes the brain sharp, which is a strict no-no when the idea is to lose your memory.

**Brain Booster**

*Even in retirement work as long as you can even if it's just part-time. Consider volunteering.*

## 56. The Morning Poison

Early in the morning, the brain is fresh. After all it had a whole night's rest. That is why morning is a good time to do

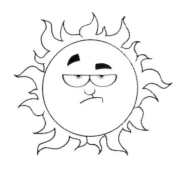

some thinking, analyzing, reading, and studying—all the intellectual stuff. Since the brain is highly active in the morning, it absorbs information at a rapid rate. But there is a great way to dull your morning-fresh brain so it does not get smarter—

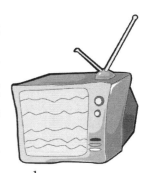

switch on the television. Listen to that one-way blabber, and soon you will feel dull and your brain will lose its morning freshness. Given thirty minutes of mindless sound pollution, your brain will feel tired before you even begin your work.

🕯️ *Brain Booster*

*Don't watch television in the morning at all. Don't even let it blare in the background. Keep noise around you to a minimum in the morning.*

## 57. Neighborhood Association Meetings

Many of us live in neighborhoods. Each neighborhood usually has a neighborhood association. These associations have regular meetings in which they discuss issues affecting your house and lifestyle. Some may argue that attending such meetings is important so you don't get blindsided by some changes you don't like. These meetings can be stressful, however. Each time you participate in such a meeting, your brain gets an opportunity to interact, analyze, and argue. It becomes smarter. But we want memory loss; we don't want a smart brain. So try to avoid all such meetings.

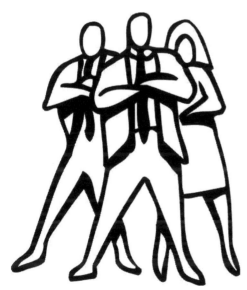

**Brain Booster**
*Attend your local neighborhood association meetings. It will protect your interests as well as your brain.*

## 58. The Non-negotiator

Let's be proud of our ability to avoid negotiations. We buy a lot of things every day. We often have time to negotiate, but we don't do it. We get lazy or afraid. We don't call our credit card company asking them to waive our late fees. We don't try to get our way with friends when deciding where and when to hang out. We just follow. No worries! Everything is cool. You are preventing your brain from developing or using negotiation skills. Soon you will become a pushover.

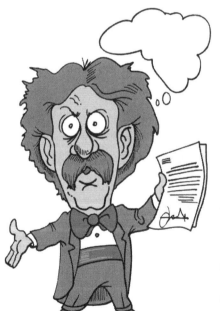

**Brain Booster**

*Negotiate the price, negotiate the place, and negotiate the time. Don't worry whether you win or lose. You will get something out of it.*

## 59. Calculator Kids

Use the calculator all the time. Never try to add, multiply, subtract, or divide mentally. You'll be surprised — your brain will shut down its calculation center forever.

Why do Chinese and Indian kids appear smarter? It's because they learn to calculate large numbers without the help of a calculator. Likely Chinese people also have lower occurrences of dementia. 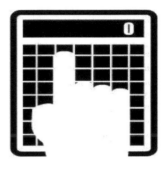 Maybe there is a connection. In developing countries many people cannot afford calculators and their schools don't allow them either. Hence they preserve the ability to do mental calculations from youth into middle age. But in developed countries we have the advantage of using calculators, which allows the brain to become dull.

*Brain Booster*

*Don't use calculators. Do calculations mentally as much as you can. Keep those number circuits whizzing in your brain. So tell me what is; 15 + 19 =?*

## 60. One Way Every Day

Lose your memory by never trying a new route. Always use the one you know. We all go to work the same way every day. We don't change it no matter what. Someone might tell us about a shorter and better route, and we are surprised we didn't know about it. People who try new things—such as taking a different route to work or the mall—do not easily develop memory loss. New things stimulate brain cells and become stronger. In order to lose your memory, stick to the habit of driving the same road every day. How do you tell it's not stimulating your brain cells? If you drive to work and don't even notice the roads then you're heading straight toward downtown dementia.

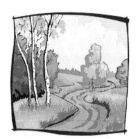

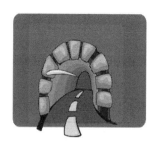

*Brain Booster*

*Find new ways to get to work. Change routes frequently. So what if it takes longer? Start a little early. Try to avoid using GPS. Use it only if you get lost.*

## 61. Mum in the Meeting

We all have to go to those boring meetings. We must go in order to keep our jobs. But what difference does it make whether we say something in the meeting or not? What if we say something wrong? To make a comment in the meeting is a lot of work. The brain has to gather courage, think of what to say, analyze how it might be received, and then say it in time before the meeting moves on to the next topic. All you need to do is to keep mum in the meetings—it's a good way for the brain to become dull and unproductive. That should aid in memory loss for sure.

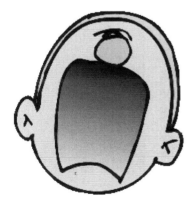

**Brain Booster**

*If you are forced to attend meetings, participate in them. Don't waste your time keeping quiet.*

# 62. Responsible for Nothing

Never take a position of power or great responsibility. Do not take over a project or a team. Because if you do,

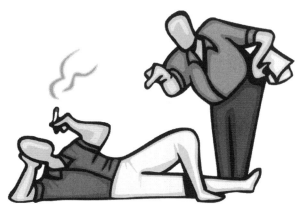

you will have to make sure the project is successful. Otherwise you will lose face or even lose your job. Moreover if you do accept responsibility, then your brain will have to work harder to avoid any negative consequences. If you get into the habit of assuming responsibilities, it's unlikely that you'll ever lose your memory. This also includes responsibilities at home, such as taking care of the neighbor's kids or pets, agreeing to do taxes, and so forth.

*Brain Booster*

*Assume more responsibility than you think you can handle. You will be surprised.*

## 63. No Further Questions, Your Honor

Curiosity kills. As kids we're controlled by curiosity. We ask questions and look for answers; we become richer with knowledge. As we grow older, the brain suppresses curiosity. It tries to get us to accept norms and stop asking silly questions.

Wherever you are, whatever you're doing, whomever you are talking to—do not make the mistake of asking questions. Just suppress your curiosity and move on. If you ask questions, you will get answers, and your brain will run faster and smoother. Not a good idea!

*Brain Booster*
*Be curious. Ask questions.*

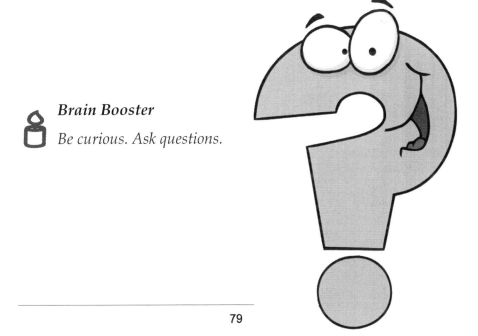

# 64. Shopping Spree on the Same Tree

Do not find new shopping places. If you know one or two places, look no further. Suppress the urge to discover other shopping gems hidden in the city. Only shop in the major chain stores. They are all set up the same way and carry the same items in the same aisles. Your brain will not have to work very hard to find merchandise in the store. Your brain will never have to navigate new stores and different setups. That's one of the reasons chain stores are successful — people like to shop in familiar environments. That's because the brain is lazy about learning new things. It doesn't want to go through the rigors of becoming familiar with a new setup. Help the brain with this phobia of shopping in new places, and destroy your memory.

 *Brain Booster*

*Do shop at local independent businesses. Help both the local economy and your brain.*

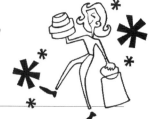

## 65. Car Wash at the Car Wash

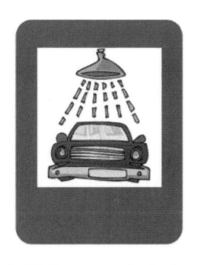

Do you wash your car at home, or do you drive to an automatic car wash? Washing the car yourself at home is exercise, and exercise prevents memory loss. It is also mental work. While you wash, the lazy brain tries to find the quickest and easiest way to finish the task. All that thinking causes a lot of brain cell stimulation. Such activity will prevent you from getting those defective brain cells that proudly associate themselves with memory loss. So drive to the nearest automatic car wash, and never wash your car at home.

**Brain Booster**

*Try to wash your car at home instead of using the automatic car wash. It could be fun and stimulating in many ways. Wink!*

## 66. Pessimistically Yours

If you're not already doing it, this strategy can affect several spheres of your life and lead you to an unexciting life. Be a pure and dedicated pessimist. Not only will you turn people off so that they stop seeing you, but it will also become a self-fulfilling prophecy. Soon you will find yourself socially isolated and depressed. And we know depressed people don't exercise their brains. They lose the motivation to do anything. Nothing new happens in their lives, and their minds become dull. Memory loss then scavenges on whatever is left.

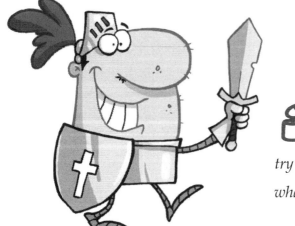

*Brain Booster*

*Be optimistic. Always try to find the positive in whatever life throws at you.*

## 67. I Am Not Joking!

Never ever tell jokes. People who tell jokes are popular among their friends, family, and colleagues. Telling jokes is not that easy. First of all you either have to be creative and make up funny stories, or you have to remember the jokes you've heard or read before. Then your brain has to figure out the best way to deliver the joke to get the most laughs. Also the attention you get after telling a good joke is a nutrient for your brain. Oh, those brain cells love attention. Once they get attention, they crave it even more. They work harder to get more attention and become smarter in the process. So just keep your mouth shut, and try not to tell any jokes. You will become boring, and people will avoid you. You can then twiddle your thumbs in your golden years.

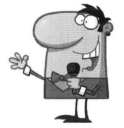

 *Brain Booster*

*Become a fun person. Tell jokes – original or not.*

## 68. LOL: Laugh Only a Little

Laughing is dangerous for our goals. Did you not hear about the guy in India who has a laughing club? Members of the laughing club get together every weekend for an hour to laugh. Yes! They just go and laugh for a whole hour. Laughing can make you happy and relaxed. It can make your brain more efficient. People are attracted to people who are happy and laughing. Then you end up with so much human

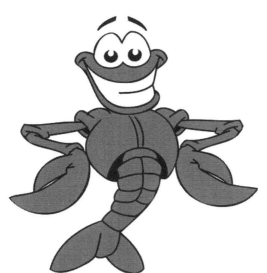

interaction that you may fall off the Dementia Express wagon. Just can your happy feelings and don't laugh—you will soon forget how to.

*Brain Booster*

*As we get older, some of us forget to laugh. Train yourself to laugh again. Funny, eh? Why are you not laughing?*

## 69. The Chef Without a Recipe

Why are you cooking? Stop cooking now. You have enough money that you can afford to go out and eat or get something delivered. Cooking is a great, relaxing exercise for the brain cells. The brain has to use at least three sensory signal inputs— vision, smell, and taste—to make cooking work. Since getting food is the most important function for the brain, as we discussed in the introduction, the brain is always very meticulous when it comes to cooking. So once you stop cooking, your cooking skill memory will slowly fade away. You will lose yet 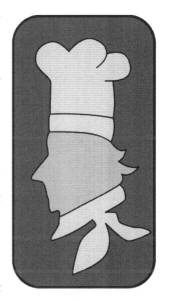 another function of the brain. This seemingly insignificant loss of skill will one day lead to memory loss.

🕯 *Brain Booster*

*Cook most of your own meals. If you don't usually cook, try to do it more often.*

## 70. The Procrastinator

Have you observed that people who stay on top of their to-do lists don't usually lose their memory in old age? They stay sharp. It's probably because they don't procrastinate. As a result they are always involved in some kind of activity that builds brain power. We need to avoid that. When we procrastinate, the brain slowly steers us toward activities in which it doesn't have to work—activities such as watching television or going to sleep early. The brain does not like to work unless you make it work. Your brain will thank you if you give it memory loss because then it does not have to work. Period.

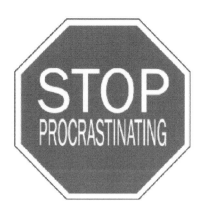

*Brain Booster*

*Do not procrastinate. If you have something on your to-do list, then do it.*

# 71. Help, It's the Rubik's Cube

Destroy all Rubik's Cubes. Rubik's Cube is one of the most intimidating puzzles ever made. The brain is initially attracted to the bright colors on the cubes. But then after playing it for a little while, the brain realizes it will take too much time and energy to solve it. No wonder the cube then gathers dust under the sofa for rest of its lifespan. After a few days, even looking at the cube causes a headache.

But we are not just talking about Rubik's cube. We are talking about all other puzzles, such as crosswords, Sudoku,

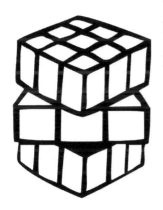
and the like. These puzzles make the brain sharper and have been proven to prevent memory loss. Be very careful.

*Brain Booster*

*Solve the Rubik's Cube at least a few times in your life until you are comfortable with it.*

## 72. Don't Shop Around — Just Shop

Never research prices or quality when you go to buy stuff. Many times we go to the store, see something we need, and buy it. Too much money in the pockets must be preventing us from thinking. Or is it the brain? We should do the same with big-ticket items as well. We don't need to take the time and effort required to find the store that offers the best price. We rather just pay a few hundred bucks extra and get it over with. Just buy it. Don't even think about searching for a better price or brand. Who cares?

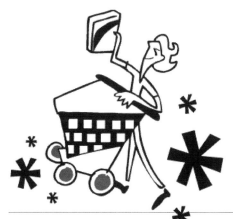

**Brain Booster**

*For big-ticket items search online and offline for a better price. You will save money and exercise your brain.*

# 73. It's a Lonely Life

Make yourself a loner. I have already offered several tips on how to make you less appealing to other people. Don't laugh, don't smile, don't tell jokes, be pessimistic, don't socialize, don't go to parties, and don't make small talk. If you practice these habits, you will soon become a loner, and your brain will not be able to practice its communication skills. Soon these communication skills will become defective, and you will accelerate toward the world of memory loss.

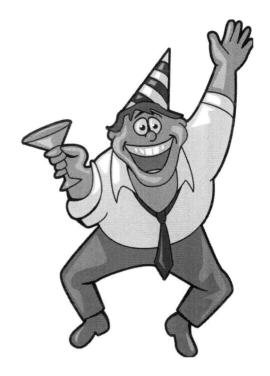

 *Brain Booster*

*It's worth repeating: be an optimistic, funny socializing junkie.*

## 74. Mary and I or Mary and Me

We don't have to worry about losing our handwriting skills as typing becomes the dominant method of writing. Technology helps kill the writing center of the brain. But there are other smart-people habits that won't let us have memory loss. When smart people write or type, they are very careful about grammar, punctuation, spelling, and so forth. We all learn these things in school, but if we stop practicing our writing skills, we'll eventually lose them. We forget calculus because we never use it after finishing school; likewise we forget the periodic table of elements. Similarly if you stop practicing good grammar, you'll forget it too.

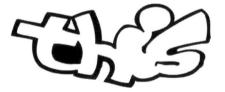

*Brain Booster*

*Be careful about your grammar and spelling, whether writing by hand or typing, or even speaking.*

## 75. How to Create Nothing from Nothing

Creativity is the enemy of memory loss because it makes the brain work very hard. That's not good at all for those who want dementia. The more people attempt to be creative, the more creative they become. The more intelligent the brain becomes, the more it explores new venues to unlock creativity. In the process it learns new things. Creativity is addictive. The satisfaction of creating something new is a tonic for brain cells. The reward cycle pushes the brain toward intelligence, not dullness. You shouldn't even try to be creative if your goal is memory loss.

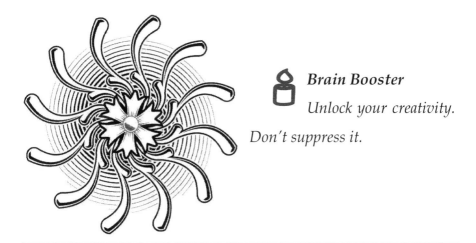

**Brain Booster**
*Unlock your creativity. Don't suppress it.*

## 76. I Don't Feel Good

If you are depressed, then memory loss will come easily. Depression leads to a lack of interest in exercise and other activities. It also leads to decreased socializing. It causes unhappiness and a lack of motivation. Depression can cause sleeplessness and weight gain as well. Depression is a great recipe for memory loss unless you intervene by seeking treatment from your doctor. If you do nothing, you'll lose your memory over the years.

*Brain Booster*

*If you feel depressed most of the time, or you are not interested in any activities, then talk to your doctor. Maybe you have depression. There are medicines that can help you.*

# 77. Technology Is for Geeks

If you have not learned to use a computer, you don't have to. If you don't know how to connect the cables from your Blu-ray and DVD players to your television, you are doing just fine. You won't miss your memory once you lose it. You won't even know.

Why do the kids in every household know exactly how to operate the remote control, but the adults struggle with it? If kids can do it, adults should be able to do it as well. Is that not logical? But the brain hates learning new 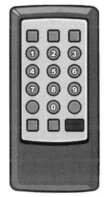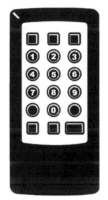 things. If it keeps learning new things, then it will not lose its memory, which is actually the brain's dream retirement.

*Brain Booster*

*Learn to connect and operate the electronics around your house. If your kids can do it you should be able to do it too.*

## 78. My Way without the Highway

Highways are scary places and it is better to avoid them. Cars whiz by at breakneck speeds, change lanes, exit, and so on. We have to dodge all this and get to our destination. On the highway the brain has to make split-

second decisions to avoid accidents and keep up. The unsuspecting brain gets a lot of exercise on the highway. You've probably noticed that the more you drive, the less you have to think. That's a sign of your brain becoming more efficient by learning skills. If you want to lose your memory, avoid the highways. Be afraid of them, and soon you will lose the skills needed to drive on the highway.

*Brain Booster*

*Drive on the highways. Simple activities like driving will help prevent memory loss.*

# 79. Dancing in My Dreams

Never dance if you want to lose your memory and dull your brain. Dancing is for monkeys. Research has shown that ballroom dancing prevents memory loss. Dancing involves a lot of steps, coordination of movement, coordination with music, and split-second error correction. These activities can make the brain sharper. That's not what we want, right? We should just be happy watching *Dancing with the Stars* on television.

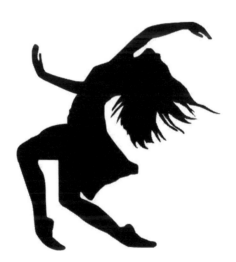

 *Brain Booster*
*Learn to dance, and dance for life.*

# 80. Board Games Are Vintage

All these board games people play only lead to excessive thinking. Strategizing, socializing, communicating, etc., are all involved in board games such as chess, monopoly, and the like. Don't you see that those elderly folks who play board games in parks or coffee shops are sharp street smarts? Playing these games guards them against memory loss. As long as you don't join them, you'll be fine.

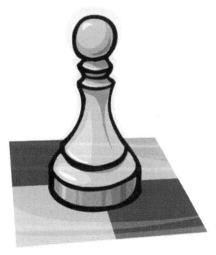

**Brain Booster**

*Play board games. Learn chess and play it regularly. It is a fun way of spending an evening with your family.*

# 81. Video Games Will Ruin You

Your parents were right. It will ruin you. Research has shown that kids who play video games are smarter than kids who just watch television. The concept is simple: television is one-way communication; the brain does no work. Video

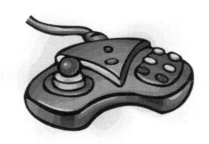

games, however, involve lively split-second interaction between the game and the brain. As more complicated games arrive on the market, even adults are lured into playing. Games such as the Wii or Kinect add physical activity to playing video games. That's an extra bonus to help the brain avoid dementia. So if you want to lose your memory, don't mess with video games.

 *Brain Booster*

*Play video games rather than watch television. I know you like this brain booster.* ☺

# 82. Don't Daydream

Don't daydream! Use that time to watch television or lie down listless on the couch. Daydreaming spurs creativity in the brain. And if you daydream about something and become passionate about it, then you might end up pursuing the dream. In the process of pursuing the dream, you will learn and do many creative things that will ruin your chances of losing your memory.

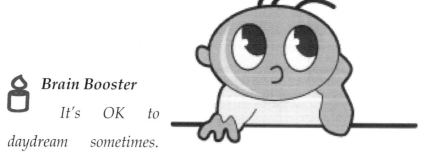

*Brain Booster*

*It's OK to daydream sometimes. Let your imagination take you places.*

## 83. Be Very Afraid

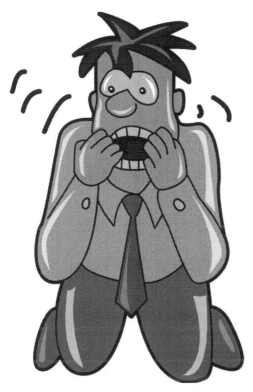

Fear is an emotion. Most of the time, it doesn't really mean anything. But you should give it great importance. Cultivate fear in yourself. Fear is a valuable tool for your brain to avoid work. If you want to do something, all your brain has to do is invoke fear to prevent you from doing whatever it is. You might not want to cross the hanging bridge. You might be scared of flying. Conquered fear is a vitamin that rejuvenates the brain. Befriend fear and you will miss out on many activities that can prevent memory loss.

 *Brain Booster*

*If you can't be fearless, at least don't be fearful.*

# 84. Logs in the River of Life

Do not be like the people who try to do their homework and make a life of their own. Be like those who flow in the river of life and let life decide what happens to them. The first types are more successful and brainy since their brain has struggled to figure out how to become successful. The latter kind did not use their brain as much. Don't worry they can sometimes become successful by chance, but because their brains have mostly rested throughout life, they're more likely to experience memory loss and a dulled mind.

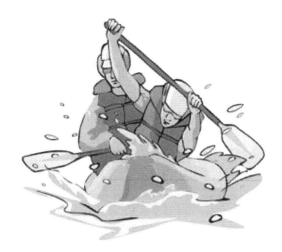

 *Brain Booster*

*Decide where you'll go in life, and act to get the life you want.*

## 85. No More School

To lose our memory, we should avoid all kinds of classes or exams. School is tough on all of us. We yearn for the day we don't have to learn anymore. And once school is over, we detest any kind of class or exam. Consequently our ability to learn and take tests decreases. Without realizing it we suddenly find we can never be students again. People who don't immerse themselves in perpetual learning have more chance of losing their memory.

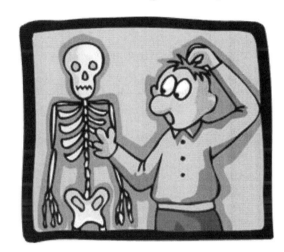

🕯️ *Brain Booster*

*Take a class — maybe photography or some kind of continuing education course. Take an exam, such as the GMAT or GRE.*

## 86. Goal? What? When? Where?

There's a big problem with setting a goal for oneself. Once you decide to achieve something, your brain has to instantly start figuring out how to do it. While you're at it, hurdles arise and your brain has to toil to overcome them. Achieving the goal gives you sense of satisfaction and a boost in self-esteem. Repeat the pattern, and you end up with a highly active brain. So don't set any goals, then your brain doesn't have to work that hard. What? You already set some goals before reading his book. Don't worry. Just pretend these goals are not important, and don't try to achieve them. Once you fail you will get frustrated and lose your self-esteem. These negative feelings are toxic for your brain and will make it dull and unmotivated.

*Brain Booster*

*Start by setting small goals and accomplishing them. Then push toward bigger goals. Maintain a pattern of establishing and achieving goals in your life.*

## 87. Find It on the Map? Why?

Do you know where Bulgaria is on the map? Or Minnesota ? Don't worry if you don't—that just means you're like most other people. As long as you know where your house is, what difference does it make? Such ignorance also boosts your chances of losing your memory. It's like a magic potion for memory loss.

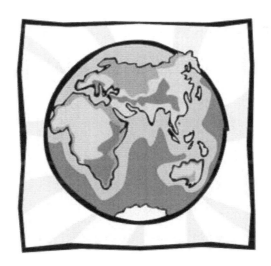

*Brain Booster*

*Know your geography. Read the atlas and know where other countries and cities are. You might get inspired to visit them.*

# 88. The Conversation Tuner

Do you sometimes just tune out a conversation because you're not interested or you don't understand it? You do? 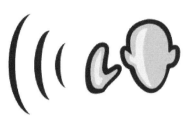 Perfect! This way you can be in the classroom yet not absorb an ounce of information. Your brain will love this lack of participation since it doesn't require much 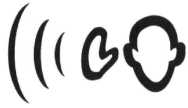 work. And the brain will grow weaker and meeker. Soon it will become a habit, and you'll have to consciously make an effort to participate in conversation. This reflex of tuning out conversations will have impact many years later in the form of memory loss.

🕯 *Brain Booster*

*Don't tune out conversations. Try to participate in them. Remember, other people can notice when you are not listening even on the phone.*

## 89. Never Wonder Why

Curiosity is never good. People who are curious ask a lot of questions. If they can't find the answer, they read, research, and try to get to the bottom of the mystery. If they still don't find the answer, they start thinking and hypothesizing. That's how most inventions and discoveries are realized. That's the reason people such as Einstein and Newton never got memory loss. Their brains were active until the very end. We're not going to be like them, correct? We will try not to be curious so we can deprive the brain of this source of rejuvenation.

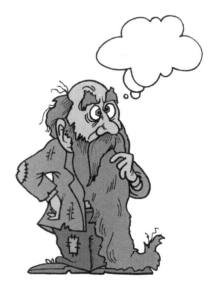

*Brain Booster*

*Be curious. Be inquisitive. Don't suppress your inner voice asking questions. You will get new ideas.*

# 90. Abstinence

Sex is the most popular physical activity, yet many do not have sex even once a week. After all you are busy running around making money and stressing out about everything. Sex and orgasm are known to have relaxing effects on the brain. It is almost like rebooting the brain. In addition you have to figure out a lot of things during sex, like how to please your partner and how to top your previous performance. These considerations force the brain to make swift decisions during sex. So if you want memory loss and a slow brain, do what most people do — avoid sex.

*Brain Booster*

No candle here;)

# 91. No Teasing Zone

Banter among family and friends is healthy for the brain. Teasing requires quick rebuttals and fast reflexes from the brain. For you to get memory loss, you need to avoid teasing and banter.

Exposure to healthy teasing and banter will also increase your self esteem and ability to handle awkard situations. Do not let your brain get that efficient. Always feel offended when you are the subject of teasing, and discourage it in others around you.

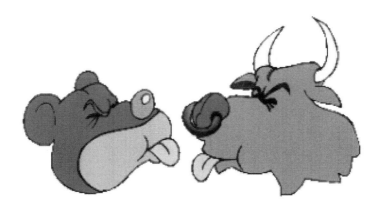

 ***Brain Booster***
*Healthy teasing and banter are good.*

## 92. B$_{12}$? Is That an Airplane?

Did you know that vitamin B$_{12}$ deficiency is a reversible cause of memory loss? Your brain needs B$_{12}$ to function. In people who do not have the ability to absorb vitamin B$_{12}$, the brain does not function normally. Once the condition becomes chronic, they get full-fledged memory loss. So if you want full-blown memory loss, do not get your B$_{12}$ level checked. Vitamin B$_{12}$ is so powerful that if someone has memory loss due to a deficiency, giving him or her a vitamin B$_{12}$ injection can reverse it.

Some of the signs of vitamin B$_{12}$ is burning of the feet, fatigue and anemia. Doctors usually do not check its levels in most patients. Some patients may have inherent genetic deficiency.

*Brain Booster*

*Ask your doctor to check your vitamin B$_{12}$ levels. Some people do not absorb Vitamin B$_{12}$ from their stomach into the bloodstream. They will need injections as pills won't work for them.*

## 93. Protection? From Who?

Using condoms prevents sexually transmitted diseases such as HIV and syphilis. Untreated HIV can cause memory loss called HIV related dementia; once it happens it is not treatable. Syphilis has three stages. The third stage is called *neurosyphilis* and affects the brain in a very gruesome way. Neurosyphilis starts showing its symptoms ten to twenty years after contracting syphilis. Patients experience memory loss in this stage. Fortunately treatment with penicillin may improve it to some extent.

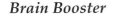 *Brain Booster*

*Use condoms to prevent sexually transmitted diseases and be monogamous.*

# 94. The Honeymoon Is Over

Even though we all enjoyed flirting when we were young, do not flirt anymore. Flirting requires a lot of mental energy. What is the other person thinking? How do you get his or her attention? Who do you get advice from? Should you approach the person? Many other questions might arise. What a great exercise for the brain, even though the questions might seem trivial after a few years. If you are married, get rid of the desire or the energy to flirt with your own spouse. Stop making him or her happy. Stop surprising each other. Then you won't be using your brain cells as much Likewise if you're single and in your forties or fifties and do not flirt at all, you will dull your brain. If you don't do anything about it, soon you will be without a social life, without energy, without a spouse, and without memory.

*Brain Booster*

*Be free to flirt, no matter how old you are. If you are married, flirt with your spouse. Cook some love.*

## 95. The Bag of Problems

Life is full of problems we have to overcome every day. Gravitate toward solving the simple problems in life. Avoid more complicated problems. For the complicated issues you've yet to tackle, the brain has to perform more complex calculations to find solutions.

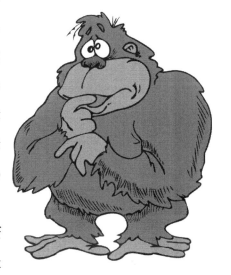

Due to its inherent laziness, the brain resists recruiting these higher centers. That's why our first instinct is to quit when we fail; we want to just skip the problem and jump to something else.

The brain knows that if it does engage in complex problem solving, then it will have to increase its efficiency. That means retirement for the brain — a.k.a. memory loss — will be pushed further away.

**Brain Booster**

*When you face problems, solve the most complicated ones first. The easy stuff usually takes care of itself.*

## 96. Cats and Dogs

Never keep pets. Pets are great friends to humans. When we have pets, we have to take care of them. Taking care of somebody delays memory loss because the brain realizes it has to keep up with somebody else's needs. You've surely observed that people's minds often start to deteriorate after their kids move away from home.

I once took care of a parrot for four days as a favor to my neighbor. I was amazed how a six inch bird kept a six foot human on his toes. I was running back and forth to make sure Mr. Parrot is comfortable. It was a pleasure too. And a great exercise for the brain. But you do not fall into the trap. Stay away from pets.

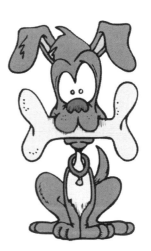

*Brain Booster*

*Keep a pet. Cats are easier to take care of than dogs but dogs will make sure you get some exercise too. You chose.*

## 97. Have We Met Before?

Do not ever attempt to register the names and faces of new people you meet. The lazy brain gives us a good reason: once I am done with this new creature in front of me, I'll probably never need him again. Why should we waste precious memory space in the neurons to register his name? If we do end up meeting this stranger again, so what? Such ignorance allows the brain to reduce the amount of work it does to what is necessary. This keeps a limit on what the brain can be asked to do. And if you let the brain succeed in this treachery, you'll have memory loss at your doorstep.

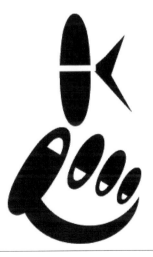

### ⚲ *Brain Booster*

*Try to remember the names and faces of people you meet. It will not only improve your memory but also make you popular.*

## 98. Wow, That Was Fast!

If you have never played racquetball, I strongly suggest you never step into the court alone or with a friend. If you did, I guarantee you won't be able to see the ball flying across the court for the first couple days. But continue to play every day, and soon your brain will be able to track the high-speed ball all over the court. In addition your reaction time will become a lot faster. Such is the elasticity of the brain. If you force it to do something, it will get better at it every single day. Oh, I almost forgot—you're reading this book so you can lose your memory. So don't play fast-paced games.

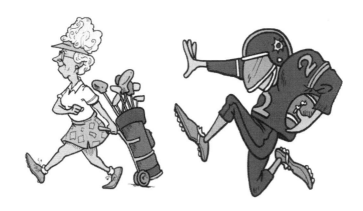

*Brain Booster*

*Don't just focus on slow games such as golf or chess. Try some faster ones too, such as badminton, racquetball, or ping-pong.*

## 99. No Hablo French

Learning a foreign language is overrated even though our world is becoming global. People travel and do business in other countries in different languages. This is leading to broad cross-cultural exchanges. Students are learning new languages. Once upon a time it was hip to learn French, Spanish, and now Chinese. But be careful. Research shows that the more languages you know, the less likely you are to develop memory loss. So if you do not need an interpreter in Timbuktu, you most likely will not be able to taste the wonder-less world of memory loss. And you cannot unlearn a language. So you have to strive not to learn one. After all why would you even need it?

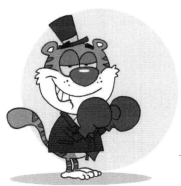

### Brain Booster

*Learn a new language. Practice it by talking to native speakers. Teach your kids more than one language. It will help them too.*

## 100.  Dumbfounded and Spellbound

Be very afraid. Turn down any opportunity to speak in public. Do not even try. What if something happens to you? Who will read this book?

Do you think the biggest fear people have is death? No! For most people the biggest fear is public speaking. I don't know about animals, but maybe they fear public speaking as well. This fear works for the brain because 99 percent of people do not speak in public. That means 99 percent of us are listeners only. Most of us fear public speaking to some degree. So you have two choices: either go against this fear and speak publicly until the fear is gone, or succumb to it and never speak on the stage. If you decide to go for public speaking, let it be clear that your chances of losing your memory will diminish. Don't blame me for that later. Public speaking involves thinking about the topic and managing nervousness. You also have to consider expressions, gestures, posture, and other factors. This is so much work that the brain devised fear as a method to prevent us from speaking in public. Public speaking rarely kills anyone, yet most people prefer death to public speaking.

## Brain Booster

*Public speaking is a very safe activity. Become a speaker.*

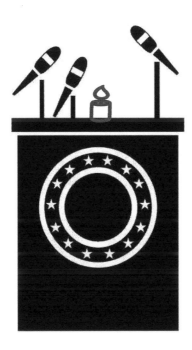

Psst…where is the brain booster candle? Look carefully. That is where you should be. ;)

11509019R00073

Made in the USA
San Bernardino, CA
20 May 2014